IBS Symptoms Can Be Managed With Diet

Discover A Collection Of Satisfying Recipes For Ibs

Antoinette M. Odom

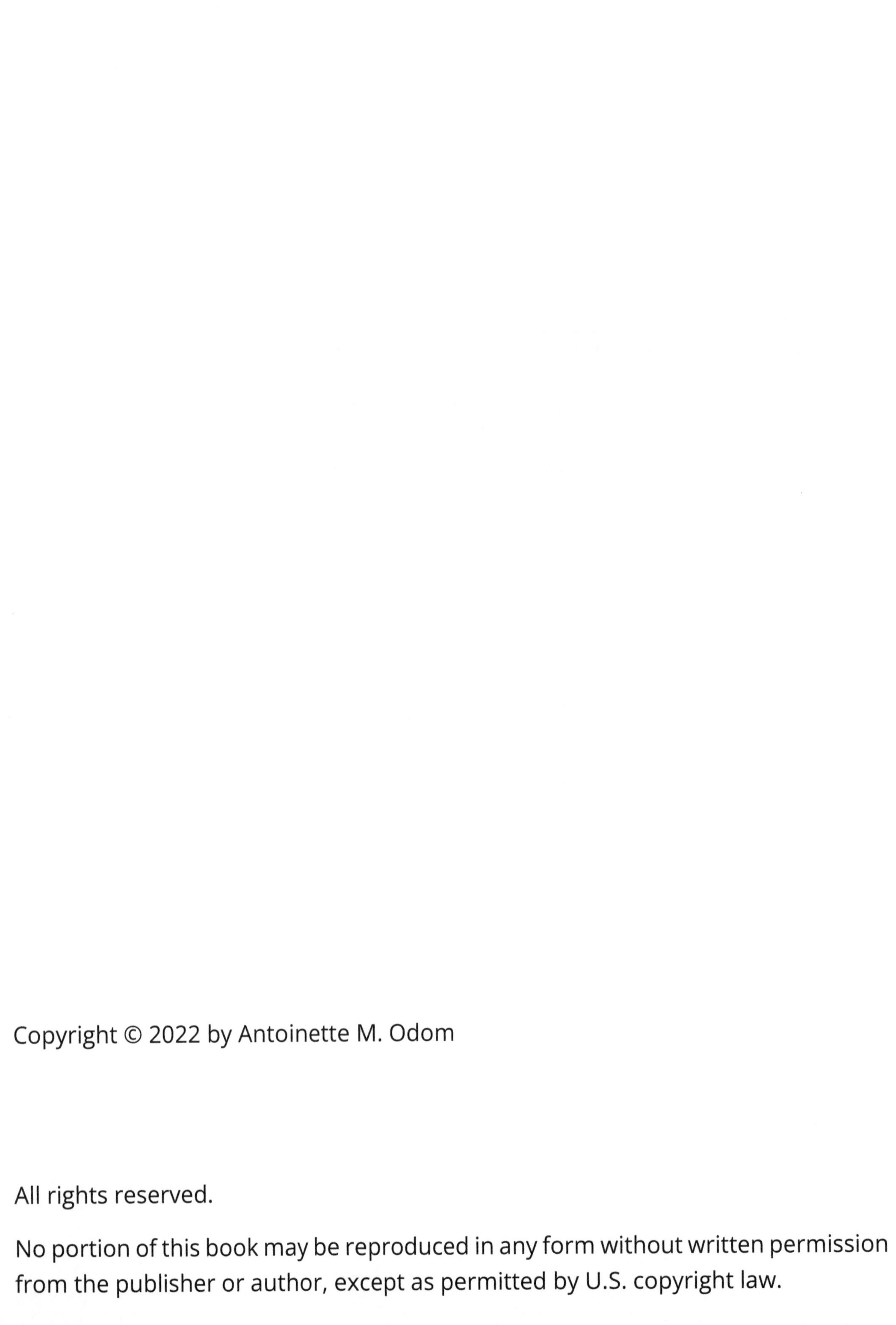

Contents

Chapter 1

Introduction

Researchers at Monash University in Melbourne developed the FODMAP diet, which they then put to the test in real-world settings. Professor Peter Gibson and Susan Shepherd of Monash University in Melbourne are the pioneers of the low-FODMAP diet. Prof. Dr. Sue Shepherd is a board-certified advanced accredited practicing dietitian and a board-certified advanced accredited nutrition professional. The treatment of food biases is a focus of her professional life. The Alfred and Monash Universities in Australia are home to Peter Gibson, who is a teacher and supervisor of gastroenterology. He was formerly a teacher of medicine and head of the Eastern Health Clinical School in the United Kingdom. Essentially, a FODMAP-limited diet is a way of eating that eliminates certain foods from your diet for around 2 months and a half. Consider certain veggies, natural goods, wheat, and dairy products, to name a few examples.

Research into the Food Map

In recent years, a rising number of scientific research from across the globe have shown that lowering FODMAPs in the diet may help lessen symptoms in persons who have irritable bowel syndrome (IBS) or other functional bowel disorders (FGA). In contrast to popular belief, the FODMAP diet is supported by scientific evidence and is becoming more popular across the world. Logic has established, for example, that a low FODMAP diet is beneficial in alleviating the symptoms of Crohn's disease in the United Kingdom (76 percent of members accomplished side effect control). A study was recently conducted at Martini Hospital in Groningen with 30 patients with IBS who had been selected by their main care physician. The participants were selected by their primary care physician. Every member of the group was required adhere to the eating plan religiously for six months. High FODMAP foods were reintroduced into the diet in order to achieve this goal. The nutritionists at the clinic provided guidance to the patients in this regard. Following the eating regimen resulted in less complaints from no less than 73 percent of the 30 patients. After a second round of introduction, it was discovered that lactose, polyols (carbohydrates seen as occurring in, for example, cabbages, vegetables, and sugars), and fructans (carbohydrates found in leafy foods) were all sensitive to the organism's presence. Several patients abruptly left the facility, claiming that the feeding regimen was inconvenient. In addition to the fact that it has been shown in several studies in various countries, the researchers are certain that the FODMAP diet is an effective therapy for a large number of patients suffering with bad-tempered entrail condition.

Following that, there's something more, as well as other investigations to look into.

To begin, let us define Fodmaps.

A supplement (particle) that might induce stomach grumblings such as gas formation and stomach anguish is known as FODMAPs. The nutrients are short-chain carbohydrates and related alcohols, including oligosaccharides of fructose (fructans) and galactose (galactans), disaccharides (lactose), monosaccharides (fructose), and sugar alcohols (polyols) such as sorbitol, mannitol, xylitol, and maltitol. Short-chain carbohydrates include fructans, galact These supplements are either inefficient or not digested in the tiny digestive system, and they end up in the large intestine as waste.

IBS, intestinal symptoms, and spastic intestine

FODMAP carbohydrates are insufficiently consumed by everyone. Everything that is not absorbed by the small intestine is sent to the interior organs. The starches are instantly developed or turned over by the gastrointestinal bacteria that are present in the environment where they are consumed. When chemicals and gases are produced, the digestive system grows in size as a result of this. The result is an enlarged tendency and fart in those who have sensitive digestion organs (spastic digestive system, IBS). These sugars may also pull in moisture from the digestive system, causing the digestive system to swell and expand. In response to the stress, you experience abdominal swelling as well as agonizing pains. Lactose (milk sugar), fructose (natural product sugar), and carbohydrates from grains such as wheat, cabbage, and beans are examples of these starches, as are other sugars.

How common is irritable bowel syndrome? How many individuals suffer from it?

It is estimated that 15 to 20% of women and 5 to 20% of men suffer with Irritable Bowel Syndrome (PDS) in the general Dutch population (calculated based on self-revealing). According to the Centers for Disease Control and Prevention, the rate in daily practice (CMR) has been 2 to 3 per 1000 people per year in males and 6 to 7 per 1000 people per year in women between 1998 and 2006. It is 4 for every 1000 males and 10 for every 1000 females in terms of commonness (as measured by the commonness index). PDS is projected to have a global preponderance of 14 to 24 percent in females and 5 to 19 percent in males, according to current estimates. Thus, almost 2 million Dutch citizens are dissatisfied with their government. It has been shown that the FODMAP diet is effective in treating IBS in a large number of people. The evidence, according to researchers, is between between 50 and 85 percent conclusive. Assuming you were correct, the FODMAP diet would be beneficial to 1 million Dutch people!

FODMAPs are naturally occurring carbohydrates that are present in the foods we consume on a daily basis and help to form the foundation of a healthy diet.

It is an abbreviation for F Fermentable Organic Degradable Polyols and Polyols

Oligosaccharides are a kind of sugar (fructans and galactans). D Disaccharides are sugars that are not metabolized by the body but rather by the liver (lactose).

These may be found in dairy products such as cheese and yogurt. Strictly speaking, monosaccharides (M) are a kind of carbohydrate (fructose).

Foods that are high in chlorophyll are good sources of this. Polyols with the letters A and P in them (sugar alcohols).

Sugars, fruits, and vegetables contain these compounds.

In the tiny digestive tract, FODMAPs are little atoms (starches) that are ineffectively or not digested, and hence end up in the internal organ. The colon is home to a diverse collection of bacteria.. FODMAPs are fermented (= eaten) by the bacteria in a short period of time and in large amounts. This causes symptoms such as bloating and flatulence, which are caused by the gas being released. Because more fluid is drawn to the small and large intestines, symptoms such as diarrhea and irregular bowel motions might occur. If you avoid consuming foods that have a high concentration of FODMAPs in your diet, you will allow fewer of these atoms to reach your colon. The same cannot be said for everyone who is easily irritated. When it comes to practicality, little amounts of FODMAPs are tolerated without issue.

Each of the FODMAPs has a unique function.

Every one of the FODMAPs is discussed in detail here.

The relationship between each gathering and a list of food sources that are low in FODMAPs or high in them will be obvious....

For the most part, the information on the chemical composition of FODMAPs comes from Monash University in Melbourne, Australia. Items on the rundowns may be overlooked. For example, everyday Dutch objects that they are unfamiliar with in Australia or that a poor person has been unable to repair.. For further information, see your dietitian.

Android and iPhone applications, such as the Monash University Low FODMAP Diet application, may be quite useful.

A few apps are available for those following a low FODMAP diet, however they are limited. Reliability has not been examined in depth with this.

Oligosaccharides

Most people have problems with the oligosaccharides fructans and Galatians.

Fructans

Wheat products (bread, cereals, and pasta) and a few vegetables, such as onions, are the primary sources of fructans in the diet. Inulin and fructooligosaccharides (also known as oligofructose and FOS) are two different sources of fructans that have been added as prebiotics to several low-fat yogurts and milk beverages, as well as to certain dietary fiber arrangements. Inulin is used in the food industry as a product enhancer in products such as skimmed milk and other dairy products. fructans are incapable of being broken down by anybody. Due to the fact that the overwhelming majority of people consume a large amount of fructans, they are most likely the primary cause of IBS symptoms. They may be found in a variety of food kinds, as well as in large quantities in our food supply, including meat and poultry. Listed below are goods that are low in fructan as well as high in fructan.

Galactans

Galactans, also known as galactooligosaccharides (GOS), are most often found in food as the sugars raffinose and stachyose, among other things. Hemp seeds, kidney beans, lentils, and chickpeas are all good sources of fiber. Individuals with IBS may have a variety of symptoms because galactans, like fructans, cannot be metabolized or ingested by them.

On this page, you will find a list of items that contain low levels of galactan and products that have high levels of galactan.

Disaccharides

Lactose is the only disaccharide in food that may behave as a FODMAP.

Lactose

Cattle's milk, sheep's milk, and goat's milk all contain lactose in naturally occurring quantities. It is extremely possible that lactose will be digested when it is separated in the small digestive tract by the enzyme lactase. Lactase is found in the bulk of the small intestine, where it works as a digesting enzyme. Lactose malabsorption occurs as a result of a shortage of this protein, and the objections that occur as a result of this are referred to as lactose bias. Depending on factors such as nationality (people of Asian origin often produce less lactase) and the presence or absence of certain digestive disorders, the amount of lactase catalysts produced by a person might vary. There is no such thing as a lactose-free diet; instead, we've compiled a list of goods that are low in lactose while yet being high in lactose..

Monosaccharides

The fructose monosaccharide is the most major monosaccharide that may act as a FODMAP in foods.

Fructose

Foods containing large levels of fructose, also known as organic product sugar, may be found in large quantities in a variety of food kinds, notably in leafy greens. It is also used as a sugar in a variety of culinary products, as well as to enhance the look or surface of food products. Fructose bigotry is the term used to describe how an excess of fructose might trigger PDS symptoms in certain people. They are not required to abstain from fructose (or any other organic substance) on an ongoing basis. Fructose may be consumed in small amounts without causing symptoms of PDS as long as the fructose is compensated by glucose or the diet contains more glucose than fructose is present.

To get the most out of organic products, it is better to nibble on a little portion of the proper sorts of organic products many times during the day rather than eating the whole thing at once. We've put up a list of goods that are low in fructose and high in fructose.

Polyols

Sugars, known as polyols, are insufficiently ingested by a significant number of people. They are referred to as polyols and include sugar alcohols such as sorbitol, mannitol, maltitol, and xylitol, among other ingredients. Normal occurrences of these contaminants have been observed in some natural goods, notably stone natural items, as well as certain plants. When used as humectants (substances that retain moisture) and imitation sugars, they are often found in foods such as chewing gum, peppermint, and sweets that are labeled "no sugar added." Polyols may be distinguished by their E numbers when used as a sugar substitute: sorbitol (E420), mannitol (E421), maltitol (E965), and xylitol (E966), for example (E967). Additionally, according to the package, excessive usage may have a purgative effect. Additionally, the drug isomalt may have a similar effect. Goods with low polyol content and products with excessive polyol content

Those that are low in FODMAPs and foods that are high in FODMAPs are discussed.

Chapter 2

A list of foods that are low in FODMAPs and high in FODMAPs follows. Labels should be reviewed.

An object's mark contains a great deal of information about the item itself. Fixtures on things manufactured by others must be reported by the maker. With the exception of combinations of green foods, all fixings should be reported in a sliding request of weight. As a result, the earlier a fixing is mentioned, the bigger the quantity of that fixing that is present in the item is. It is not harmful to consume a little amount of FODMAP. After a period of time, an item's organization may change, therefore do frequent checks for any changes.

Ingredients that should be avoided are not always easy to identify by their names. For further information, go to the list below.

Ingredients that contain FODMAPs

Oligofructose, fructose, fructose syrup, glucose fructose syrup, and fructose corn syrup are all examples of fructose-containing carbohydrates. The ingredients lactose, buttermilk, milk components, milk powder, and whey are all included.

sorbitol (E420), maltitol (E421), mannitol (E421), maltitol (E965), xylitol (E967) are polyols that are found in foods. Sorbitol (E420), mannitol (E421), maltitol (E965), xylitol (E967) are sugar alcohols that are found in foods.

IBS symptoms are triggered by FODMAPs in many ways.

Four characteristics are shared by all fructooligosaccharides (FODMAPs).

Small intestinal FODMAPs are ineffectively trapped by the body.

This means that a significant number of these FODMAP-particles are not invested in the tiny digestive system and, on second thought, end up undigested in an internal organ. There are two possible explanations for this: either they are unable to be broken down by the gut into smaller molecules, or the process is too sluggish to allow for complete absorption of all molecules while passing through the small intestine (in the case of fructose). The ability to digest and retain various FODMAPs varies from person to person - fructose consumption is delayed in all cases, regardless of genetics.

Nonetheless, some people (especially those with a brown complexion tone) progressively lose the ability to produce an appropriate number of molecules (lactase) in order for lactose to separate, and additionally, the ability to digest polyols varies from one person to another. The inability of humans to digest fructans and galactans (which are present in grains such as wheat) results in no complaints from carbohydrate sources that can be easily handled, such as sucrose (table sugar) and glucose.

Foods high in fructose and other simple sugars (FODMAPs) are small atoms that may be found in large quantities in our diet. Osmotic pressure is created when a large number of microscopic particles are present in the small digestive system, which causes them to pull in water. Additional liquid in the gastrointestinal system may create the runs, increase discomfort by increasing the amount of liquid in the system, and have an impact on muscle growth in the intestine.

A source of nutrition for the tiny organisms that ordinarily reside in the colon, FODMAPs are found in fruits, vegetables, grains, and legumes.

It is possible that atoms will end up in an internal organ if they are not picked up by the tiny digestive tract first. There are several bacteria in the colon that are there by default. The microorganisms that dwell there feed on these atoms and swiftly separate them, resulting in the production of the gases hydrogen, carbon dioxide, and methane, among others.

'Aging,' you may say. A fart, tooting, feeling unpleasant, or anguish in the mid-region are all possible outcomes of this gas production process. In individuals with PDS, a strain increase in the sensitive digestive system is most likely to blame for the aggravating objections they have.

Another possibility is that the production of gas (methane gas) might postpone the growth of food deposits in the colon in certain persons, hence contributing to the obstruction. If the sugar chain of the molecules is short, they ferment more rapidly than long molecules such as oligosaccharides and sugars. When compared to dietary fibers, short sugar chains ferment more quickly than long sugar chains.

Cumulative effects are felt by everybody.

FODMAPs may be found in a variety of forms in a single supper meal. Because they all induce comparable digestive system protests once they reach the bottom section of the small digestive system and colon, their possessions have been grouped together for ease of identification. In this case, the combined effects of all individual FODMAPs must be considered. This kind of complaint is based on the total amount of FODMAPs consumed (or tanked) each meal, rather than the total amount of FODMAPs consumed by each type of FODMAPs. When someone who has difficulty digesting both lactose and fructose consumes a meal that contains a small amount of all FODMAPs (lactose, fructans, polyols, galactans, fructose), the effect on the intestines is 1 + 1 + 1 + 1 = 5 times greater than if he or she had consumed or drunk the same amount of only one of these FODMAPs. While changing one's diet, it is important to keep track of the total amount of FODMAPs present in one's meals.

Using the FODMAPlimited diet, it is possible to reduce the amount of gas and fluid that accumulates in the digestive organs by eating smaller portions more evenly spaced throughout the day and by consuming less FODMAPs in general.

Where does the PDS come from if we don't all have it.

What is it about eating FODMAPs and producing gas that causes one person to get PDS while the other does not? It is possible that this is being done for five different reasons.

When it comes to how much gas we generate, This is dependent on the kind of bacteria that exist in the digestive tracts as well as how they handle the gas produced by the stomach. Almost every human has a unique mix of microscopic organisms in his or her digestive system, and certain microbes are more active fermenters (gas formers) than others in their digestive tracts.

The digestive tracts have an innate feeling. There are some people who have more fragile gastrointestinal systems than others. Whether we feel sick or not depends on how much our digestive tract's sensory system changes: how much of our digestive tract's sensory system changes before we begin to feel uncomfortable. Grumblings are only experienced by those who have a sensitive stomach after ingesting an excessive amount of FODMAPs in one sitting.

Once the digestive system has been properly formed, how effectively it can expel gas will be measured. When a large amount of gas is produced, the gastrointestinal system is generally activated, causing the gas to be swiftly moved through the digestive organs until it is expelled as a breeze as soon as possible. Despite this, gas may accumulate in the digestive organs of certain people who have IBS, resulting in a more severe amount of stomach distension in some individuals.

Which organs of digestion are most responsive to being enlarged. When our digestive organs are properly configured, our muscular strength contracts for the most part, preventing our mid-region from expanding. It is natural for the stomach (a large muscle located underneath the lungs) to unwind throughout the process of establishing the digestive system. This unwinding allows greater room in the abdomen for the digestive organs. It should be noted, however, that these reflex reactions are weak in some persons who suffer from IBS. Digestive distension may cause constriction and smoothing of the stomach, which causes the midsection to be pushed forward and (in female patients) to seem pregnant when used in conjunction with certain medications. As an added bonus, this creates a significant amount of frustration.

Our sensitivity to signals from the digestive tracts, as well as our response to these signals Our ability to regulate signals from the digestive tracts in an unexpected manner is enhanced under more favorable circumstances. Pressure and events in our life have an influence on our ability to distinguish. Stress and weakness might cause the digestive systems to become more vulnerable. The functioning of the 'cerebrum-gastrointestinal axis' is further enhanced as a result of this.

to look into it

In recent years, a rising number of scientific research from across the globe have shown that lowering FODMAPs in the diet may help lessen symptoms in persons who have irritable bowel syndrome (IBS) or other functional bowel disorders (FGA). In contrast to popular belief, the FODMAP diet is supported by scientific evidence and is becoming more popular worldwide. Taking as an example, a scientific report focused in the United Kingdom indicated that a reduced FODMAP diet is beneficial in lowering symptoms of IBS (76 percent of members accomplished side effect control). Thirty individuals with IBS were selected by their primary care physicians for a study conducted at the Martini Hospital in Groningen in 2014. Sixty-two months of strict adherence to the diet were required of the assembly. It was in this manner that high-FODMAP foods were once again introduced into the diet. Medical clinic dietitians guided the patients through their nutritional needs and preferences. Following the eating regimen resulted in less complaints from no less than 73 percent of the patients. Extreme sensitivities to lactose, polyols (starches present in foods such as cabbages, vegetables, and sweets) and fructans (carbohydrates found in leafy foods) were discovered during a second round of administration. In a hurry, two patients left, claiming that the eating regimen was causing them discomfort. Furthermore, based on findings from other nations' study, the experts are certain that the FODMAP diet is an effective therapy option for a large number of persons suffering with crabby intestine disease.

Chapter 3

Problems with the digestive system

What about you? Do your digestive organs give you problems, and do you have the impression that food is the source of your problems? If this is the case, it is usually beneficial to investigate whether drugs or foods are to blame for the problem in question. Many people who suffer from gastrointestinal problems suffer from the unpleasant side effects of farting or swelling, which are caused by an excessive amount of gasses in the digestive tracts on a consistent basis. By using atoms that have not been absorbed, colon bacteria produce gas. Fermentation is the name given to this cycle.

Fats, proteins, carbohydrates, nutrients, and minerals are all included in our daily diet.. Numerous carbohydrates, such as dietary fiber, are poorly digested and do not absorb well in the small intestine. Unlike dissolvable dietary fiber, insoluble dietary fiber cannot be matured (eating) by bacteria in the stomach, but dissolvable dietary fiber may be aged (eating) by stomach microorganisms Some single short-chain sugars (oligosaccharides) and sugar alcohols are also poisonous and cannot be digested by the stomach, but are instead broken down into gases by the stomach microbes.

Do you too suffer from the negative consequences of gases and farts on a daily basis? Eat less carbohydrates; otherwise, your complaints may escalate to a higher degree of intensity. It is beneficial to identify which carbohydrates are causing your symptoms in order to keep them at bay.

Gingival bacteria help to age the short-chain sugars and carbohydrates that many people suffering from digestive problems are exposed to on a daily basis (the inexpensive food for the microorganisms). The FODMAPs are a group of short-chain carbohydrates that are harmful to our health. Aside from gas and farting, FODMAPs may also produce loose bowels, discomfort, cramps, and constipation in some individuals.

All people have poor retention of fructooligosaccharides (FODS). Those FODMAPs that do not pass through the small intestine are absorbed into the internal organ system. The starches are promptly aged or transformed by the digesting tiny organisms that are readily accessible in such environment. As a result, chemicals and gases are produced, resulting in the expansion of the digestive system. People with sensitive digestive systems (spastic stomach, PDS) may have a swollen inclination and tooting as a result of this.

These sugars may also pull in moisture from the digestive tract, causing the digestive system to swell and expand. The result of the stress is a bloated stomach and severe discomfort. Lactose (milk sugar), fructose (organic product sugar), and carbohydrates from grains such as wheat, cabbage, and beans are examples of these starches, as are other sugars.

FODMAP is a short for fructooligosaccharide-containing oligosaccharide-containing oligosaccharide-containing oligosaccharide-containing oligosaccharide-containing oligosaccharide-containing oligosaccharide-containing oligosaccharide-containing oligosaccharide-containing oligosaccharide-containing oligosaccharide-containing oligosacc

If you decide to follow the fodmap diet, you should be certain that your symptoms are caused by IBS and not by another illness. Therefore, we recommend that you consult with your primary care physician before commencing the dietary regimen.

Elimination and reintroduction stages are included in the fodmap diet.

In general, the low FODMAP diet is divided into two sections: the disposal diet, which is followed by a reintroduction phase, which is used to determine what is causing the symptoms. The rules recommend that you stick to a consistent eating routine for a long period of time in order to significantly reduce your exposure to FODMAP-rich foods. This plethora of carbs is initially eliminated from the diet for approximately one month, depending on the individual. Because it is a very strict dietary regimen, consulting with a dietician is everything from a wasted expense. Numerous people report significant relief from their objections during this so-called "end phase. " It is authorized to include an accumulation of sweets into the eating routine at all times throughout the following several weeks. Fruit sugars (apples, mangos, honey) and dairy sugars (cream, cheese) are examples of carbohydrates (milk, yogurt). If and when the objections reappear, it is immediately apparent who is to blame. In the following days, you return to your fundamental diet and experiment with a new carbohydrate. Finally, you have a diet that is tailored to your needs and does not include any of the carbohydrates that you dislike. In order to avoid grumblings, you should stick to your dietary routine. When it comes to how much FODMAP a person may tolerate before experiencing symptoms, it varies from one person to another. It is critical to restart the introduction of FODMAPs into the cycle. Dietitians, preferably those who specialize in gastrointestinal nutrition, should be consulted in order to follow the recommended eating plan. When it comes to how much FODMAP a person may tolerate before experiencing symptoms, every individual is unique.

This interaction is fundamentally dependent on the introduction of FODMAPs in a new and improved way. Dietitians, preferably those who specialize in gastrointestinal nutrition, should be consulted in order to follow the recommended eating plan. How much FODMAP admission can be tolerated before side effects begin to manifest depends on the particular individual. This interaction is fundamentally dependent on the introduction of FODMAPs in a new and improved way. A dietitian, preferably one who specializes in gastrointestinal nutrition, should be consulted before beginning the eating regimen.

Guidance from a dietitian

Trying to follow a low-FODMAP diet is not easy. Although the eating regimen is not new, not all dietitians and general experts are familiar with it. Therefore, it may be necessary to observe a dietitian who is familiar with the eating regimen in question. Several food types high in FODMAPs should be avoided prior to entering the first stage (disposal stage), according to the dietitian who will advise on this. Individuals who adhere to the eating plan will return to the dietician after a period of severe low FODMAP restriction. In the words of the registered dietitian:

It determines how well you respond to dietary restrictions and how resistant you are to them.

Ensures that you get enough variety in your diet and that you don’t get any wholesome deficiencies (in the long run).

Assists with understanding marks and how to manage social gatherings and eating out

Reduced-Fodmap Consumption during the festive season if possible

The low-FODMAP diet has been shown to cause issues with special occasions, such as weddings and birthday celebrations, in many people who adhere to it. The possibility that “mistakes” will be made is a source of concern for many people.

To understand that there is no prejudice or sensitivity associated with the low FODMAP diet is critical. In other words, you can withstand specific food sources in specific quantities. One of the problems with party menus is that many ingredients are combined in small amounts, and that the menu is frequently supplemented by excessive alcohol consumption.

The following are some suggestions for navigating the holidays without incident: Is it your own profession to be a host or an entertainer? After that, you can prepare a FODMAP-friendly menu for your family on your own time. Suppose we bet that no one will come to the house and look around.

Whether you’ll be dining with friends or family, you should decide beforehand. Make it clear to the host or group leader that you are serious about ensuring dietary modifications are implemented. Consider offering to bring something yourself if you believe they will have difficulty changing specific items. For example, you could make the soup and prepare a desert on your own.

To avoid disappointment when dining out, inform the establishment ahead of time that you will not be able to consume all of the food options and whether they will be able to provide substitutes.

Because only one out of every eight gourmet specialists is aware of the FODMAP-poor diet, you may want to make some suggestions of your own.

APERITIF SUGGESTIONS FOR MENUS

Although one glass of dry (shimmering) white wine, cava, prosecco, or champagne is permitted, there are a variety of non-alcoholic alternatives to choose from, such as:

Cranberry juice and spray water are served as an aperitif. Lime or lemon juice can be added to water.

Cucumber and lemon infused water

Spritz water with ginger or ginger syrup infusion (be sure to check the label for fructose content!).

DRINK WITH APERITIF SNACKS

Crackers made from buckwheat and quinoa are used in place of toast.

Toss the crackers in a bowl with a tapenade of green or black olives and serve immediately.

Chips that are salty.

Use caviar or fake caviar to decorate crackers after they have been dipped in egg.

Siege crackers topped with smoked fish (salmon, halibut, trout), arugula, and capers

Raw vegetables should be served as follows: carrots should be cut into strips, cocktail tomatoes should be placed in a pot, and chicory leaves should be laid out on a saucer. Dip the vegetables in the dressing before serving them (mayonnaise or cocktail sauce that you make yourself by adding mayonnaise with some tomato puree).

Cucumber and hard cheese, or cherry tomato and mozzarella, on a skewer are two options. Using rice sheets as the base, create mini quiches and fill them with artichoke hearts.

It is important to exercise caution when using wraps because they frequently contain polyols (for example, E422), which can cause health issues in some people.

SOUP

To make soup, omit the onion and garlic from the recipe.

The ingredients for purchased soups are typically onion and garlic; the ingredients can be found on the ingredient list of the product.

Onion is a common ingredient in soup vegetables. Buy pre-sliced soup vegetables if that's something that interests you. Then opt for a non-mixed variety, such as celeriac or broccoli florets, rather than a mix of vegetables (in the cooler compartment).

Use the green parts of spring onions and wild garlic to make this dish. Only a small amount of the green part of the leek is used (80 grams per portion).

Make use of other flavors instead of bouillon cubes, such as fresh thyme or fresh herbs, to give your dish a unique flavor boost (watercress, parsley). Make use of your cream to finish the soup: instead of traditional cream, use soy cream, rice cream, oat cream, or another vegetable-based cream alternative to finish.

DISHES FOR THE PRIMARY PARTY

Make a selection from the list of vegetables that are permitted. Look for a method of preparation that does not include the addition of sauce, stock cubes, or a combination of vegetable herbs. Steamed or stewed vegetables that have been season with salt, pepper, and fresh herbs are the most flavorful options.

Aside from marinated or breaded preparations, meat, poultry, and fish are not considered to be a problem.

Cooking with onions and garlic is a must when making game stews, stew meat, or hare ragout.

Buckwheat pasta, rice noodles, or buckwheat-based pasta can be substituted for wheat pasta. Gluten-free pastas are available in a variety of flavors.

Specify that you want the sauce to be served on the side.

DESSERT

Sorbet

Ice cream made from soy beans Ice cream made with coconut.

Merengue is a dessert that is made from whipped egg whites and sugar, and it is served chilled. You can eat it plain or make a pie crust out of it, and you can top it with fresh fruit if you want to (permitted varieties).

Salad de fruits selon les variétés de fruits permises

DRINKS

It is recommended that you drink water, spray water, or flavor water.

Various types of teas are available, including black tea, white and green tea, fruit tea made from the fruits that are permitted for consumption, Chai tea, dandelion tea, peppermint tea, Rooibos tea, and rosehip tea. Consume the tea in reasonable quantities and avoid letting it sit for too long.

It is best to keep alcohol consumption under control. Colas and other non-alcoholic beverages

Caffeine-free coffee should be consumed.

You can still enjoy the holidays if you plan ahead of time.

THE 3 DIET PHASES: The Elimination Diet (also known as the elimination diet) This stage lasts approximately one month, during which time you will eliminate all high FODMAP food varieties from your diet. The evaluation of your manifestations will take place one month after they have begun. Is there any progress? It's possible that the eating plan isn't the best option for you if this is the case. Should it improve, proceed with the following steps:

Finally, it's time for the big show! In this section, you will incorporate specific items from the FODMAP collections into your diet while also keeping track of any symptoms you may be experiencing. As a result, you have a list of foods that you are able to consume as well as those that you are unable to consume. As soon as you've done that, you're in the game:

It is possible to live a low-FODMAP diet. In the eating routine, this is the final period to be consumed. Know which items make you feel uncomfortable and avoid them at all costs! If you have any leftover FODMAPs, they will be remembered for your next meal plan. Last but not least, this last section is critical. Because it is detrimental to continue to be in the disposal stage for an extended period of time, it is best to move on. In most cases, disposal slims down are prohibitively expensive, and it is attempting to meet your dietary supplement and fiber requirements. It is not reasonable to have a deficiency in vitamins or fiber for your health. Please do not allow yourself to be placed in this situation!

It is critical in the FODMAP lifestyle to retest yourself for your food responsive qualities on a regular basis, just like clockwork. You can count on your stomach to restore itself on its own timetable, and the microbes in your stomach, as well as your stomach health, are constantly changing. A food touchiness that you currently have may not be available in 90 days if the manufacturer does not make it at this time. Suppose you never tried again in the future and never discovered that you were able to eat specific food varieties again! That would be a shame!

Products with a Low and a High Fodmap

When it comes to understanding the foods that you can and cannot consume, these rundowns are invaluable.

The identity of the person responsible for the rundown isn't always clear, and is the information reliable?

Typically, the rundowns are out of date; when was the last time one was updated?

If you have a rundown that has been written or printed on paper, it is not difficult to find a specific item.

Fodmap Products - The Most Comprehensive List Available

When following the Low FODMAP Diet, it is recommended that you use the Low FODMAP Diet application, which is available for both Android and Apple devices. Whenever the college attempts a new item, this application is refreshed, and it provides you with information on low FODMAP foods as well as information on segment size. In this way, you always have a reliable source of information about FODMAP in your pocket when you need it.

A traffic signal system is utilized by the application. Green foods are those that can be consumed indefinitely.

Every feast in the specified amounts can be supplemented with 1 orange item per 1 item of each feast. Items in the color red should be avoided at all costs!

This method will assist you in selecting the items that are most appropriate for you and your preferences.

Products containing a high level of FODMAP

Consider the following list of items from the high FODMAP starch groups as an illustration: 1.

Produce such as vegetables and legumes is available.

The following vegetables: garlic, onion, artichoke, asparagus, and celery

vegetables such as: fresh beets, black-eyed peas (beans), cauliflower, celery root, falafel, sauerkraut (e.g. sour), lentils, and lentil soup

vegetables such as leek, mushroom, and peas

cured vegetables; savoy cabbage; soy beans; green onions; Shallot

The fruits apples, apricots, avocado; bananas, ripe; blackberry; sweet cherry; dates; feijoa; figs; grapefruit; guava; mango; nectarines, peaches, pears, peaches and pears persimmon; dried pineapple; prunes raisins; sea buckthorn; canned natural products; watermelon.

Chapter 4

Meat sausages Chorizo.

Grains and cereals; bread and cookies; pasta; nuts and cakes; and other baked goods; Products containing wheat, such as cookies, including chocolate-covered cookies; wheat bread; and other baked goods.

breadcrumbs;

Cookies, muffins, and croissants made with wheat-based cereal.

donuts

noodle soup with egg;

Several types of cupcakes are available.

More than 1/2 cup cooked pasta made from wheat;

Bran, wheat cereals, and wheat flour are all examples of grains that are commonly used in baking.

Wheat germ; wheat noodles; wheat rolls; wheat cereal

Bread:

cereal bran; couscous, granola, cereal muesli; roasted pistachios; rye crackers; Semolina; almond flour; amaranth flour; barley, including flour; rye crackers; Semolina

Sauce, sweets, sweeteners and spreads made with agave; fructose; sauce if it contains onions; corn syrup; seasonings, sauces, sweets, sweeteners and spreads

The following items are included: hummus honey; jam; strawberry jam; molasses; pesto; and quince paste.

sucrose-free confectionery

the pasta made with tahini

E numbers for sweeteners and the sweeteners they correspond to:

acacia gum; isomalt (E953 / 953); lactitol (E966 / 966); maltitol (E965 / 965); mannitol (E241 / 421); sorbitol (E420); xylitol (E967 / 967); acacia gum

Medicinal plants that contain prebiotics

Yoghurts, bars, and snacks can all be disguised with the following ingredients: The acronym FOS stands for fructooligosaccharides; inulin is a polysaccharide that helps the body absorb nutrients.

oligofructose.

Coffee, tea, and protein powders are all options.

a variety of fruit and herbal teas, including chamomile, fennel, and dandelion; large quantities of fruit juices; a chocolate-flavored malt beverage;

HFCS soda, meal replacement drinks containing milk-based products, and sports drinks are examples of such products.

Lactose-containing foods Sour cream; yogurt; kefir; buttermilk; cheeses, cream; ricotta custard; sour cream; yogurt; kefir; buttermilk;

Icing on the cake

a list of low-FODMAP foods

Keeping track of calories on a low FODMAP diet can be difficult; however, this list of high-quality food sources makes it much simpler.

Alfalfa, vegetables, and beans

sprouted beans; canned and pickled beets; black beans - 45 grams

1 cup: Bok Choi; 1/2 cup broccoli (total); 2 Brussels sprouts (total); zucchini; ordinary and red cabbage (total); carrot; petiole celery (total: 20 gr); chicory leaves; chickpeas (total: 1/4 cup).

chilli;

12 ear of corn; 1/2 ear of zucchini; cucumber; eggplant; dill; green pepper; ginger; leek leaves; lentils - in small amounts;

salad: ice mass; radicchio; romaine; olives; parsnip; peas (5 pods); cured gherkins; potatoes; pumpkin; radicchio; green onions; kelp/nori; chard; spinach; sun-dried tomatoes (4 computers); swede; tomato - canned, cherry, common; turnip

Fruits

bananas, unripe, blueberries, cranberries (1 tablespoon), pitahaya, lingonberry, grapes, guava, ripe, melon, kiwi, lemon, including lemon juice, lime, including lime juice, mandarin, orange, passion fruit, papaya, pineapple, raspberry; ripe bananas, unripe bananas, blueberries, cranberries (1 tablespoon), pitahaya, lingonberry, grapes, gu

rhubarb;

Strawberry.

Foods containing animal products (meat, poultry, and substitutes)

beef;

chicken;

Kangaroo, lamb, pork, and prosciutto are some of the meats that can be found in Australia.

Ham and turkey breasts are served with mashed potatoes. Tuna in a can (fish and seafood)

Cod, haddock, flounder, salmon, trout, and tuna are examples of fresh fish.

Seafood:

crustacean (crab, lobster);

Oysters, mollusks, and shrimp are all examples of seafood.

Cereals, bread, treats, pasta, nuts, and cakes are just a few of the foods available to consumers. Bakery that specializes in gluten-free products:

Corn, oats, rice, almonds (a maximum of 15 per serving), shortbread cookies (a maximum of 1 per serving), Brazil nut

Boiled bulgur (quarter cup; 44 g); buckwheat; buckwheat flour; cornmeal (optional);

a half cup of corn flakes; coconut milk, cream, pulp; corn tortillas (3 tortillas); toasted hazelnuts

nut macadamias (maximum of 15 per person);

oatmeal (1/2 cup); millet (1/2 cup); peanuts (1/2 cup); quinoa (1/2 cup);

15 pecans are allowed; 15 pine nuts are permitted; polenta is permitted.

Popcorn, cereals, and oatmeal; potato flour; pretzels; pasta - up to 1/2 cup; Basmati brown rice; and other foods.

Noodles made of white rice, rice flour, and seeds.

The following foods are included: chia, hemp, poppy seeds; pumpkins; sesame seeds; sunflower seeds; walnuts

Seasonings, sauces, desserts, sweeteners, and spreads are all examples of products that fall under this category.

the artificial sweetener aspartame; the artificial sweetener acesulfame K; the almond oil; the capers in vinegar; the salted capers; the artificial sweetener acesulfame K; and the artificial sweetener acesulfame K;

DARK chocolate (three squares), milk chocolate (three squares), and white chocolate (three squares); Dijon mustard; erythritol (E968/ 968); fish sauce; golden syrup; glucose; glycerin (E422/422); strawberry jam / jelly; vanilla extract;

maple syrup, confiture, and other similar terms

miso paste; pesto sauce (less than 1 tablespoon); peanut butter; rice malt syrup; saccharin; hot chili sauce (about 1 teaspoon); stevia;

a sweetener known as sucralose; sugar, also known as sucrose; tomato sauce (two 13-gram bags), vinegar

L.; 2 tablespoons apple cider vinegar

1 cup balsamic vinegar, 2 tablespoons rice wine vinegar, 1 tablespoon vasaabi, 1 tablespoon Worcestershire sauce

Coffee, tea, and protein powders are all options.

Because alcohol is a digestive tract aggravator, it is recommended that admission be limited to: one bottle of beer

vodka, gin, whiskey, one glass of wine, coffee, and a snack are all acceptable.

kvass;

in small quantities; lemonade; limoncello;

Powdered protein sources include egg white, pea protein (up to 20 grams), rice protein, and whey protein isolate.

protein isolate made from whey (also known as whey protein).

In small amounts, soft drinks, such as diet cola, should be consumed because aspartame and acesulfame K can be irritating; tea: in small amounts, black tea should be consumed.

green; the color black

a mixture of mint, white, and water

Butter made from dairy and eggs

Brie and Camembert are two types of cheese.

Cheddar cheese

feta; Mozzarella; Parmesan; ricotta - 2 tablespoons; Swiss; eggs; milk; almond extract

Hemp is a type of plant that can be grown in a variety of ways, including:

dairy-free milk; macadamia nuts; oatmeal - 30 mL; rice - up to 200 mL

250 milliliters; sorbet

Weekly menu plan: 7 days a week Dietary Guidelines Based on the Fodmap Protocol

A 7-day low FODMAP diet plan is a dietary arrangement that assists you in temporarily eliminating FODMAPs from your diet, which has been shown to be a contributing factor to crabby inside syndrome (CIS).

Morning meal on the first day of the week

An unripe banana is blended with frozen strawberries, flax seeds, almond milk, and green tea to create a refreshing beverage.

Lunch

1 cup cooked earthy colored rice with baked salmon and low FODMAP vegetables (for fiber).

Dinner

Salad de printemps fraîche Choosy eaters should stick to a maximum of three vegetables (from the rundown), with protein and green onions thrown in whenever possible.

2nd day's breakfast: 1/2 cup rolled oats with water or non-dairy milk, followed by a 12 green banana.

Lunch

Shrimp Vegetarian Roast with Brown Rice Noodles

Dinner

Recipe for Risotto with Pumpkin and Carrot

oatmeal with green bananas and chocolate for breakfast on day three

Lunch Quinoa with a chicken leg and parmesan cheese, low FODMAP vegetables, and can tomatoes

The dinner salad (lettuce, ringer pepper, tomato, hay sprouts, prepared with sauce) and a cup of frail dark tea are both served.

Afternoon snack on Day 4

2 whole eggs, 1 cup rolled oats, and a shot of black espresso

Served with brown rice and roasted chicken with green onions and sunflower oil for lunch.

Dinner Romaine salad with 120 grams of barbecued chicken and a cleaved hard-boiled egg dressed in olive oil

Morning meal on Day 5

Espresso, three whole eggs, and 85 grams of ham are the ingredients for this dish.

Lunch

With eggplant and mint tea, 170 grams of charbroiled fish

a 12-cup pot of steaming earthy colored rice, 120 g of barbecued chicken with coleslaw, and a dessert

Morning meal on the sixth day

2 whole eggs, 1 slice of gluten-free bread, 60 g sharp cheddar (toasted)

Sandwiches Braised hamburger with parsnips for lunch

Meal: 170 g barbecued pork hack served with a vegetable serving of mixed greens dressed with vinegar dressing.

omelette with cheddar, chile pepper, spinach, olives and tomatoes, gluten-free toast and coffee on Day 7 Breakfast

With a glass of lemonade and a lunch sandwich made with gluten-free bread, turkey, Swiss cheese, horse feed grows, and horse feed grains.

Cooked cod with ringer pepper and 170 grams of potatoes for dinner

Some examples of Fodmap Recipes are provided below.

If a person exhibits signs of food bigotry, the most effective method for determining which foods are causing these symptoms is to follow a low-calorie diet.

For your convenience, we've included some low-FODMAP meal plans to help you get started.

To the Shepherd, Lettuce Tacos with Chicken

One and a half hours (20 minutes) for preparation

Approximately 35 minutes to complete the preparation.

Ingredients

This recipe makes six portions.

Marinade made with 50 grams of achiote;

The marinade contains 1/4 cup apple vinegar.

For the marinade, clean and devein 3 pieces of guajillo chile (seedless and deveined), then soak them in water for 30 minutes. Marinade: 2 pieces of wide chili, cleaned, deveined, and seedless, and soaked in water before use

For the marinade, 3 garlic cloves

The marinade calls for 1/4 piece of white onion. for the marinade, 1/2 cup pineapple juice

salt marinade, 1 tablespoon

For the marinade, 1 tablespoon of fatty pepper the marinade will be made with 2 cloves

Marinade made with 1 tablespoon oregano

1 piece of roasted guaje tomato, to be used as a base for the sauce marinade made with 1 tablespoon cumin

3 small chicken breast cubes (boneless and skinless) cut into small cubes

olive or flax oil (one tablespoon) The French Lettuce has reached its limit. Eva

Sliced pineapple (half a pineapple) in half moon shapes coriander leaves (about 1/2 cup)

2/3 cup purple onion, finely chopped

The taste of tree chili sauce to accompany the meal In order to complement the lemon flavor,

Preparation

To make the marinade, combine the achiote, vinegar, chilies, garlic, onion, juice, salt, pepper, cloves, oregano, tomato, and cumin in a large mixing bowl until well combined and homogeneous in consistency.

Set aside 1 hour in the refrigerator with the chicken and marinade in a bowl with the shepherd's marinade.

Cook the chicken you marinated in a skillet with the oil over medium heat until it is done, about 15 minutes. Ensure that you are adequately protected (cover).

Turn your barbecue to high heat and broil the pineapple until it is golden brown. Remove from the grill and cut into shapes to keep.

Set out French Lettuce Eva® sheets on a table and arrange the chicken to be shepherded, along with the pineapple, cilantro, onion, and a little sauce, and serve with lemon wedges on the side. Dietary supplements are available.

A 2,000-calorie diet provides a percentage of daily values. Calories The energy expenditure was 92.2 kcal. 4.6 percent is the percentage of

23 g (or 7.4 percent) of carbohydrate calories

The amount of protein in this dish is 1.6 g (3.2%)

9 g/1.3 percent of the total amount of lipids

Dietary fiber: 2.9 g (or 5.8 percent of total calories).

74% of the calories come from sugars.

The amount of cholesterol in the blood is zero milligrams per deciliter.

Chapter 5

With Garbanzo Beans and Nuts in an Apple Salad

10 minutes are required for preparation. Approximately 2 minutes to prepare Ingredients

Sliced Eva Lettuce in individual serving cups. one-half cup arugula, finely chopped

1 cup of thinly sliced green apple (about 1 cup) 1/4 cup toasted chickpeas (or other legumes). walnuts (about 1/4 cup) toasted olive oil (two teaspoons) strawberries (about 1/4 cup)

seasoning with 1 tsp of salt

Pepper (a pinch) is used in this recipe.

Recipe Preparation - 3 tablespoons of raspberry vinegar

In a large mixing bowl, combine the lettuce, arugula, green apple, chickpeas, and pecans. Toss well to combine the flavors. Completely smooth blend. Reservation.

Pour into a blender and blend until smooth. Stir in the strawberry, salt, pepper, and raspberry vinegar. It's a dream to combine.

On a plate, arrange the plate of mixed greens and garnish with the strawberry vinaigrette.

Enjoy

Dietary supplements are available.

In the context of a 2,000-calorie diet, the percentage of daily esteems.

878 kcal (44 percent of the recommended daily allowance) calorie

Carbohydrates: 122 g (41% of total carbohydrate consumption).

a total of 36.2 g (72% of total protein intake)

52.1 percent of the total is lipids. 34.1 g

73% of the calories come from dietary fiber (36.5 g).

50.3% of the calories come from sugar.

The amount of cholesterol in the blood is zero milligrams per deciliter.

Fajitas made on a sheet pan

Chili powder (two teaspoons) and salt to taste 2

2 tablespoons cumin powder

1 teaspoon paprika (smoked) Depending on personal preference, season with salt and black pepper

cut into thin strips 1 1/2 pounds of sirloin steak 1-inch-thick slice of green bell pepper, sliced orange bell pepper, peeled and sliced thinly 1/2 a red onion, peeled and sliced

Garlic cloves (about 4 to 5 cloves) minced Olive oil (about 3 tblsp.

Lime juice (freshly squeezed): 2 tablespoons

Prepare 6 (8-inch) flour, corn tortillas, or carb balance tortillas by heating them in the microwave.

Prepare a 425 degree Fahrenheit oven. Brush lightly with oil or coat with nonstick spray to prepare a baking sheet for use later.

Combine the bean stew powder, cumin, paprika, 2 teaspoons salt, and 2 teaspoons pepper in a small mixing bowl until well-combined and evenly distributed.

Bake in a single layer on a baking sheet that has been pre-prepared by placing the steak, bell peppers, onion, and garlic together. Carefully combine the olive oil and stew powder mixture with a gentle throw.

Place the dish under the broiler for 25 minutes, or until the steak is completely cooked through and the vegetables are crisp and fresh. lime juice should be added at the end of the cooking process.

Toss with tortillas and serve right away!

Sheet Pan Dinners are a favorite of many people. See what I mean? Look at these delicious lunches! Sheet Pan Tuscan Chicken, Sheet Pan Egg in the Hole, Breaded Pork Chop Sheet

Pan Dinner, and One Pan Balsamic Chicken are just a few of the recipes you'll find on this page..

Make a list of what you need to buy.

2 tablespoons chili powder (or equivalent)

Ground cumin, 1 teaspoon paprika, 2 tablespoons cayenne pepper Salt and black pepper are essential ingredients in this dish.

Sirloin steak weighing 1 1/2 pounds. pepper (green) 1 green bell pepper

1 red onion, 1 orange bell pepper

garlic cloves (between 4 and 5 cloves).

Olive oil (about 3 tblsp.

Lime juice (freshly squeezed): 2 teaspoons

6 flour tortillas (8-inch diameter) or carbohydrate balance

Facts about nutrition:

440 Calories per serving.

Fat calories account for 297 percent of daily calories.

51 percent of the calories come from fat. 33g of fat

carbohydrate 5g 2% of total carbohydrate

1 gram of fiber equals 4%

Nutritional Values: Sugar 1 g 1 % Protein 31g6 % Vitamin C (78.4mg) is 95 percent effective. Iron 3.7 milligrams (21 percent)

Tuscan Chicken on a Sheet Pan (Ingredients)

4 thighs of chicken, boneless and skinless 6 Roma tomatoes, quartered, 1 pound green beans, peeled and chopped

1 onion, peeled and cut into bits 1 cup Extra Virgin Olive Oil

1/3 cup Balsamic Vinegar 5 cloves Minced Garlic, to taste

1 teaspoon Dried Parsley Flakes 1 teaspoon Fresh Parsley 1 teaspoon Dried Parsley Flakes

1 teaspoon Sodium chloride

1 teaspoon freshly ground black pepper 2 tablespoons chopped parsley

Preparation:

Add the olive oil and balsamic vinegar to a mixing bowl or pitcher, along with the garlic, parsley, salt, and pepper, and mix well. Whisk it until it's completely smooth.

Place the chicken in a large zipper bag with a generous amount of the dressing and seal the bag tightly. Place the pack in a safe place and forget about it.

Cut the tomatoes in half and then in quarters. Cut the onion into chunks. Remove the green beans' closures and place them in a large zippered bag with the rest of the vegetables. Pour in the remaining dressing, then seal the pack and put it away until you're ready to use it.

Preheat the oven to 425 degrees Fahrenheit. Prepare the chicken and vegetables in a sheet container and set aside. A little amount of the marinade should be poured on top of the chicken. Cook for 25 minutes under the broiler on the stove, shaking the pan once during that time. Variations

With just a few minutes remaining in the cooking time, place slices of fresh mozzarella on the breasts of each bird. Return them to the broiler until they are completely melted.

When you remove the container from the burner, sprinkle it with 12 cup crumbled Parmesan all over the container. Allow it to settle for a couple of minutes before presenting it to guests.

Make a list of what you need to buy.

4 thighs of chicken, boneless and skinless

6 Roma tomatoes, peeled and quartered 1 pound Green Beans (cut in half)

1 onion, peeled and cut into bits 1 cup Extra Virgin Olive Oil

a third cup of balsamic vinegar 5 garlic cloves, peeled and minced

1 teaspoon dried parsley flakes (optional) salt and pepper to taste 1 teaspoon salt 1 teaspoon black pepper 2 teaspoons parsley

The following are the nutritional facts: 441 calories, 198 percent of which are from fat Fat 22 g (34 percent of the daily value) 5 g of saturated fat (31 percent of total fat)

40% of the population has high cholesterol (119mg).

Sodium (986mg) accounts for 43% of the total.

Potassium 1044mg 30 percent of the total

Carbohydrates (15 g, 5% of total calories)

3 grams of fiber is 13% of total calories.

Sugar (eight grams, nine percent)

43 g of protein (86 percent) Vitamin A 1500 International Units (30 percent) Vitamin C (26.1mg) 32 percent of the daily recommended intake Calcium 215mg 22 percent of the daily recommended intake

Iron (2.7mg/15%) is a trace element.

Ingredients for Sheet Pan Dinner with Breaded Pork Chops:

4 (8-ounce) bone-in pork chops, 3/4-inch to 1-inch thick, cooked in a skillet

2 big eggs, beaten with salt and freshly ground black pepper to taste

a quarter cup of milk

1 1/2 cups Panko bread crumbs

1 teaspoon garlic powder (optional) 2 tablespoons onion powder (optional) 1 teaspoon oregano leaves (dried)

1 teaspoon chopped parsley (dry)

1 teaspoon paprika (smoked) For the Broccoli and Apples, 1/4 cup vegetable oil is used.

2 cups steamed broccoli (1 pound chopped) 1 green apple (1 1/2-inch slices) 1/2 a purple onion, finely chopped 3 tablespoons extra-virgin olive oil 1 teaspoon brown sugar 1 tsp. rosemary leaves, dried

Depending on your preference, season with salt and black pepper

Preparation:

Prepare a 425 degree Fahrenheit oven. Prepare a baking sheet by lightly oiling it or spraying it with nonstick spray.

Season with salt and pepper to taste in a large mixing bowl and set aside. In another large mixing basin, combine broccoli, onion, apple, olive oil, earthy colored sugar, and rosemary.

Season the pork cleaves with salt and pepper to taste before grilling them.

In a large mixing basin, whisk together the eggs and milk until well combined. Mix together the Panko breadcrumbs, garlic powder and onion powder as well as the dried herbs and paprika in another large mixing bowl; season with salt and pepper to taste.

Working in batches, dip the pork chops into the egg mixture, then into the Panko mixture, squeezing to coat each piece. Repeat with the remaining chops.

Place the pork cleaves on the baking sheet that has been prepared; distribute the broccoli mixture around the pork chops.

Place in the broiler for 10-12 minutes, or until golden brown. Turn the pork slices over and continue to cook for an additional 10-12 minutes, or until the pork is completely cooked through. Serve as soon as possible.

Lists of things to buy

Pork chops (8 ounces), bone-in and 3/4-inch to 1-inch thick, prepared as directed on the package

Season with salt and freshly ground black pepper. 2 big eggs (about)

a quarter cup of milk

1 1/2 cups Panko bread crumbs

1 teaspoon garlic powder (optional) 2 tablespoons onion powder (optional) 1 teaspoon oregano leaves (dried) 1

a teaspoon of parsley (dry)

1 teaspoon paprika (smoked) For the Broccoli and Apples, 1/4 cup vegetable oil is used.

2 cups steamed broccoli (1 pound chopped) 1 green apple (1 1/2-inch slices) 1/2 a purple onion, finely chopped

Olive oil (about 3 tblsp.

1 cup granulated sugar 3 teaspoons brown sugar 1 tsp. rosemary leaves, dried

Depending on your preference, season with salt and black pepper Facts about nutrition: 4701.1 calories, 17.0 g of total fat 5.1 g of saturated fat

1.6 g of polyunsaturated fatty acids 7.6 g of monounsaturated fatty acids Cholesterol levels were 212.2 milligrams.

165.6 milligrams of sodium

15.7 grams of total carbohydrate, 1.9 grams of dietary fiber, and 899.8 milligrams of potassium

Chapter 6

Tomato-stuffed Eggplant served with Tzatziki sauce

10 minutes are required for preparation. Preparation time: 20 minutes 4 Ingredients / 4 Servings

2 medium-sized aubergines, sliced in half and lightly frayed Olive oil (about 3 tblsp.

1 finely chopped onion (about 1 cup) 3 garlic cloves, peeled and cut fine 1 teaspoon ground cinnamon powder 1 tablespoon cumin seeds, ground

1 tablespoon tomato puree (optional)

4 medium-sized cubes of tomato, sliced into quarters 1 tbsp. agave honey (or similar)

seasoning with 1 tsp of salt

Pepper (a pinch) is used in this recipe.

1/4 cup freshly squeezed lemon juice

1 bunch finely chopped parsley, to taste parsley (about half a bunch, finely chopped)

1/2 cup of soy yogurt (optional)

1 garlic clove (about)

3 tablespoons mint leaves, finely chopped 1 paprika pinch (optional)

Preparation

Preheat the broiler to 200 degrees Celsius.

Using a small pot with medium heat and a little oil, sauté the onion and garlic until translucent, then add the ground cinnamon and cumin, tomato puree, tomato, and the agave honey, and simmer for 10 minutes until the tomatoes are soft. Season to taste.

Aubergines are stuffed and loaded down with sautéed tomato, which has been cooked on a dish for 20 minutes and placed on a table. Remove the chicken from the broiler and set it aside.

In a large mixing bowl, combine the lemon juice, parsley, cucumber, yogurt, garlic, mint, and paprika. To frame the tzatziki, combine the yogurt, garlic, mint, and paprika. Until you get a uniform mixture, blend it for a while.

Serve the aubergines with the Turkish sauce and a sprinkle of pita bread or unleavened bread on top to complete the presentation.

Dietary supplements are available.

A 2,000-calorie diet provides a percentage of daily values.

60.8 kcal 3.0 percent of total calories

carbohydrate 9.7 g (3.2%) carbohydrate

Proteins 2.7 g, or 5.4 percent of the total

Lipids 2.1 g 3.2 percent of total lipids

Dietary fiber (3.2 g) accounts for 6.4 percent.

4 g sugars (4.6 percent of total sugars)

Cholesterol is 4.6 mg or 1.5 percent of total cholesterol.

Soup with Vegetables and Kale

10 minutes are required for preparation. Time required for preparation: 30 minutes 2 Servings of the Following Ingredients

2 tablespoons of extra-virgin olive oil

1/2 of a white onion, peeled and filleted 1 celery stick, cut into cubes (optional).

1 cup of finely chopped pore

1 tablespoon minced garlic, coarsely chopped 1 cup sliced mushrooms (optional)

1 cup sliced mushrooms, halved kale (about 2 cups)

1/2 bulb of fennel, sliced into sticks, 1/2 piece of fennel 4 to 6 quarts of beef broth

seasoning with 1 tsp of salt

Pepper (a pinch) is used in this recipe. a quarter cup of almonds

Preparation

Put olive oil in a medium-sized pot and heat over medium heat until the fragrance comes out of the onions and celery. Add the pore, garlic and mushrooms and continue to cook until the mushrooms begin to release juice. Finally, add the kale and fennel and continue to cook until it's mellow and fragrant. Continue to cook for an additional 5 minutes.

Fill with the meat stock and season with salt and pepper to taste. Cook until the mixture begins to boil, covering it to prevent it from evaporating completely.

Serve in a bowl, garnished with a bit fresh kale at the end and sliced almonds. Enjoy

Dietary supplements are available.

507 kcal (25 percent of total calories)

carbohydrate 65.6 g 22 percent of total carbohydrate

Proteins: 35.8 g (72% of total)

Lipids 16.3 g at a 25 percent concentration

11.9 g dietary fiber (24 percent of total)

12.5% of the calories come from sugars.

The amount of cholesterol in the blood is zero milligrams per deciliter.

Goat cheese salad topped with fried goat cheese

For 4 people, cooking time is 30 minutes. Homemade hard chunks of goat cheese served on a bed of freshly prepared mixed greens with ringer pepper

Ingredients

100 g mixed salad (optional) a single red pepper

200 g goat cheese (fresh goat cheese) (rounds) a single huge egg

frying oil for frying

one tablespoon almonds that have been finely chopped a single serving of breadcrumbs

flour on a single plate Dressing

a pinch of pepper and a pinch of salt

honey (about one spoonful) two tablespoons of lemon juice

juice Preparation: three tablespoons extra-virgin olive oil

Maintaining a cool environment for the goat cheddar will be the most easy approach of dealing with it. Separate the goat cheddar rounds into two groups (around 12 pieces). On a plate, lightly beat the egg. Separate the goat cheese pieces and mix them through the flour, next the egg, and last the breadcrumbs until well combined. Repeat the last two steps (egg and breadcrumbs) for an extra thick and fresh crust on top of it.

Heat the oil to 180 degrees and fry the balls for 1 minute, or until they are a magnificent golden brown color all over. After that, drain them on a piece of kitchen paper. Remove the seeds from the chime pepper and chop it into pieces, which you should then fry for 3 minutes in a skillet with the olive oil.

Discard the pepper and pour the baking fluid into a small bowl, mixing in the lemon juice and honey until well combined. Season with salt and pepper and set aside to cool. In a large mixing bowl, whisk together the dressing and the mixed greens. Stir in the ringer pepper and arrange on a serving platter with the grilled goat cheddar. Decorate with a few almonds if desired.

Dietary supplements are available.

358.2 calories per serving

Total fat: 20.7 g Saturated fat: 7.9 g Polyunsaturated fat: 3.5 g Monounsaturated fat: 7.9 g Total fat: 20.7 g Saturated fat: 7.9 g Cholesterol: 35.9 milligrams

163.1 milligrams of sodium

470.6 mg potassium Total Carbohydrate 33.5 g Dietary Fiber 4.7 g Sugars 21.1 g Potassium 470.6 mg

14.6 g of protein

Steamed Cod (enough for 4 servings)

Preparation time: 30 minutes

The superb protein found in cod animates digestion and serves as a structural substance for cells, muscles, catalysts, and chemicals, amongst other applications. Proteins that are essential in the prevention of desires and muscle breakdown.

Ingredients: four fish fillets (about 150 g each)

a tablespoon (four tablespoons) 2 bars of leek, lemon juice

a total of 3 tablespoons Rapeseed oil is a kind of vegetable oil produced by pressing seeds of rapeseed.

100 milliliters of vegetable broth Salt

Pepper

12 sprigs of dried thyme

a dozen bunches of parsley (10 g)

Making use of one organic lemon

2 tbsp. lemon juice should be applied to the fish filets after they have been rinsed and dried. Cut leeks into rings after they have been cleaned and washed

1 tbsp. of oil in a small saucepan over medium heat. Sauté for 2 minutes at medium heat after securing the fish with paper towel. Cook for 5- 7 minutes on a low heat, turning once, adding the remaining lemon juice and 50 mL of vegetable stock and covering with a tight fitting lid.

To prepare the leeks, boil the remaining oil in a large saucepan over medium heat for 2 minutes, seasoning with salt, pepper, and thyme, then remove from the heat and set aside. Cook the leek for 5 minutes on a low heat, with the remaining vegetable stock. Meanwhile, wash the chives and dry them well before cutting them into little rolls. Cut the lemon into quarters once it has been flushed with boiling water.

Season the fish filets and leeks with salt and pepper, arrange them on plates, and garnish with chives and lemon quarters to finish the presentation.

Calories: 226 kcal (Nutritional Fact)

Ingredients for a four-person vegetable lasagna:

legumes puy de bouillon (80 g).

olive oil (about 4 tablespoons plus a little more for sprinkling over veggies) 2 large tomatoes, coarsely diced 1 large beef heart, minced 1 clove of garlic 2 beetroots, diced

a half teaspoon of tamarind juice (soy sauce)

1 tablespoon dehydrated shallots, chopped 1 teaspoon cumin powder

400 g butternut squash, peeled and sliced thinly Slice 300 g zucchini lengthwise into fine ribbons and set aside.

Preparation:

180 degrees Celsius (broiler) Preheat the broiler to high heat (th 5-6). Pour enough water to cover the lentils in a small pan and set it aside. Cook for 10 to 15 minutes, or until the mixture is still somewhat stiff. Channeling and reserving are both important concepts.

As a result of these preparations, preheat the oil in a large pan and crush the tomato, which will serve as the base for the sauce. Add the garlic and beets, as well as the tamari, shallot, and cumin, and mix well to combine. Prepare the thick puree by adding 2 tablespoons of water and cooking it for 15 minutes on medium heat. Cook for another 5 minutes after adding the lentils to the skillet's contents and adding a little more water.

Spread half of the butternut and one-third of the zucchini in a baking dish and top with half of the lentil sauce. Bake for 30 minutes. Recreate the cycle with a layer of zucchini on top to finish it off if necessary. Cook for 45 minutes, or until the veggies are just soft, after sprinkling them with olive oil.

With parsley oil, you may make a substitution for the olive oil.

Facts about your diet

Nutritious meal with 65 calories

daily value expressed as a percentage

0.2% total fat (0.2% total fat).

Zero grams of saturated fat equals zero percent of total calories

Amount per serving: Polyunsaturated fat 0.1 grams, Monounsaturated fat 0 grams. Zero milligrams of cholesterol

There is nothing there.

The sodium level is 35 mg per one percent of the population.

Potassium (169 mg, 4% of total potassium intake).

14 percent of the total carbohydrate is 13 g.

The amount of dietary fiber is 4.4 g (17%).

3 12 g sugar

5.0% of the total protein is 2.9 g.

Vitamin A accounts for 85% of total vitamin C.

Calcium the presence of 2% iron the presence of 4%

Nutritional value for vitamin D is zero percent, whereas nutritional value for vitamin B-6 is five percent

Magnesium is 5 percent while cobalamin is 0%

Chapter 7

Ricotta cheese and walnuts in a lemon-garlic-zucchini salad.

Ingredients

basil leaves that have been freshly picked.

Lemons with Garlic

Walnuts with ricotta cheese.

Garlic, black pepper Zucchini squash

Extra virgin olive oil is a kind of olive oil that is extracted from olives that have not been tainted by a chemical process. Salt

Preparation

Remove the new items from the packaging and allow them to dry.

2 lemons (or other citrus fruits)

A total of 6 medium-sized zucchini squashes were used.

Fresh basil in a little bunch.

The zucchini's ends should be cut off using a knife. The julienne peeler (or regular peeler) slices vegetables into chopstick-like strips with the help of a spiralizer. Sprinkle salt over the contents of the strainer. Place the sifter on a plate or in a basin to collect any excess moisture. a.

Salt (around 1 teaspoon)

The lemons should be sautéed together with the shells, then transferred to a medium-sized mixing dish.

garlic should be peeled and chopped or pressed before being combined with the oil, lemon juice, and pepper in a mixing dish a.

cloves of garlic cloves of garlic cloves of garlic cloves of garlic cloves

extra virgin olive oil (around 13 cup)

dark pepper (around 12 tsp)

Heat a pan over a medium heat until it is hot to the touch. Pecans should be chopped coarsely before serving. Toss the pecans in a bowl for 2-4 minutes, stirring constantly. a dozen and a half cup of chopped walnuts

Remove the basil leaves from the stems and cut them into ribbons to use as a decorative garnish.

Remove excess water from the zucchini spaghetti by squeezing it with your hands. This should be repeated many times.

Combine the zucchini and dressing in a mixing bowl until the dressing is smooth.

Serve by arranging zucchini noodles on a platter and topping with ricotta cheese, nuts and tablespoons of salt and pepper. Garnish with basil and serve immediately if possible.

1 ricotta cheese package (15 oz)

Salad de tuna et légumes.

Ingredients

zucchini, 2 medium-sized (daintily cut)

carotenoids of moderate size (cut in matches)

bottles with tuna inside of them (every 5 ounces depleted in water) 1 carrot, 1 bunch of celery, 1 bunch of spinach (cut and chopped)

onions (about 1) (little, meagerly sliced)

fresh, level parsley (about 1 tbsp (slashed approximately) 4 pieces of lettuce (iceberg)

dressing (half a cup) (light fench) Yogurt (two tablespoons)

the clove of garlic (crushed)

curry powder (about 1 teaspoon)

Directions

Using a small pot filled with sizzling water, cook the zucchini and carrots for one minute. Cold water is channeled via a nozzle.

Put all of the ingredients for the dressing in a small bowl and season with salt and pepper to your liking.

Gently toss the zucchini and carrots in a medium-sized mixing dish together with the fish and other ingredients (fish, celery, onions, parsley, dressing).

Serve the lettuce leaves with the platter of mixed greens on top.

with arugula, potatoes, and vegetables

dressing

Ingredients

Potatoes (small) weighing 1 pound (peeled and halved)

green beans (around a pound) (cut and cut into pieces) Cauliflower (1 head): (small, cut into florets) Salad de entrée (serves 1) (torn into bite-sized pieces)

the flesh of one roasted red pepper (without seeds and roughly chopped) Yogurt (around 1 and a third cups)

the mayonnaise in three tblsp.

Approximately 2 tablespoons fresh basil (mince, extra leaves for garnish) minced chives, 2 tablespoons (finely chopped)

Parsley (about 2 tablespoons) (finely chopped)

Directions

For 15-20 minutes, boil the potatoes until they are tender in salted water that is boiling. Channel, cool, and cut your way through the crowds of people.

In a large pot of boiling salted water, cook the beans and cauliflower florets for 7-8 minutes, or until tender. Allow to cool fully after channeling and washing with icy water.

In a large mixing basin, combine the cooled potatoes, beans, and cauliflower until well combined. In a large mixing bowl, combine the salad and the pepper.

Dressing preparation: In a large mixing bowl, combine the yogurt and mayonnaise, then stir in the chopped spices and freshly ground dark pepper until well combined.

Add dressing to a platter of mixed greens, top with more basil leaves, and serve immediately.

Asparagus, cherry tomatoes, and cottage cheese are combined in a delicious salad.

Ingredients:

Two bunches of asparagus, both of which are green

150 g of cherry tomatoes (approximate weight) 1 cup cottage cheese (100 g). 30 g walnuts, peeled

Kikos (approximately 30g) (toasted corn)

peeled sunflower seeds (approximately 20 grams) Use two tablespoons of apple cider vinegar. Extra virgin olive oil (four tablespoons) Pepper and salt are two of the most important spices in cooking.

Preparation

The asparagus should be cleaned before cooking. Begin by rinsing the asparagus under a stream of cold water and cutting it into pieces of equal size. Remove the toughest piece from the stem and set aside.

Cook by bringing water to a boil. While assembling the asparagus, bring a large pot of salted water to a boil in a separate dish and cook it for 10 minutes, or until the asparagus is tender but still intact.

This is interfering with the preparation of the meals. To finish, remove them from the pan by drenching them for a couple of seconds in cold water to stop the cooking process, then set them aside. So they'll be able to maintain their extreme green coloration. In order to remove all of the water, channel them again afterward.

Prepare the other ingredients for the dish (see below). The tomatoes should be washed, dried with permeable paper, and then cut in half. Disintegrate it by channeling the curds. Cut the nuts into small pieces as well, if possible. Vinaigrette should be made first. In a large mixing bowl, combine the vinegar and salt. Then, while whisking constantly, slowly drizzle in the oil while continuing to beat with a fork until the dressing is extremely well emulsified (about 5 minutes).

Impersonate someone else and serve. Asparagus should be divided among four serving plates. In a separate bowl, combine the tomatoes, curds that have disintegrated, and pecans that have been slashed. Make a dressing out of the vinaigrette from the previous day. Finish with sunflower seeds and kikos that have been slashed to perfection.

Roasted Brussels sprouts in a creamy sauce in the oven.

600 grams of Brussels sprouts

Bacon (250 g)

Potatoes (800 gm) (floury in pieces) two hundred and twenty milliliters of milk

Just one pepperoncini with a sweet point a glob of melted butter (plural)

cheese that has been manually grated

herbs in 200 gr of cream cheese Pepper and salt are two of the most important spices in cooking.

Necessities

Approximate dimensions of the oven dish: 20 by 28 cm.

Preparation

200 degrees Fahrenheit is required for the broiler to be operational. In approximately 15 to 20 minutes, the potatoes will be ready. While waiting, cook the brussels sprouts for 10 minutes in a skillet of water, according to package directions. In a dry skillet, cook the bacon until it is firm. Then add the pointed bell pepper, cut into pieces, and mix well.

In a blender, blend the potatoes with the milk, spread, pepper, and salt until they form a puree. Drain the potatoes after crushing them finely. Combine the bacon, chile pepper, and brussels sprouts, reserving 5 or so for garnish. Combine the cream cheese and spices in a large mixing bowl until well blended. Using a baking dish, divide this mixture into sections.

Toss the potatoes in a blender and puree until smooth. The leftover Brussels sprouts should be divided down the middle and placed over the highest point on the stove dish. Place the stovetop dish under the broiler for another 20 minutes to melt the cheese and finish baking.

Alternatively, instant puree can be used for a more expedient version of this recipe.

Chapter 8

Salmon poke bowl in a bowl of rice

Ingredients

Salmon fillet (250 g) prepared fresh Avocado, if you will.

Rice (150 g): (sushi)

a dozen cucumbers, two tablespoons rice vinegar, and sesame seeds mandarin oranges 175 g

Alfalfa hay (about 30 g).

Sauce:

Mayonnaise, two tablespoons lime juice (two tablespoons) to your personal preference

Marinate the salmon in the following ingredients:

soy sauce (1 tablespoon)

Sesame oil (one tablespoon) Lime juice (about 1 tbl)

Preparation

In order to make the jab bowl, you can use both regular and sushi rice. Cut the salmon into blocks, combine with the marinade ingredients, and refrigerate for as long as possible in a shrouded container in the refrigerator. Rice should be prepared first, followed by a sprinkle of rice vinegar. Cucumber, mango, and avocado should all be cut into small chunks before eating.

In a large mixing bowl, combine all of the sauce's ingredients. Salmon, rice, cucumber, avocado, and mango are divided into discrete planes by partitioning the 3D shapes of the salmon, rice, cucumber, avocado, and mango that are north of two dishes. Horse feed, lime mayo sauce, and sesame seeds can be used to dress up the dish for presentation.

Chopped cabbage stuffed into burritos

Ingredients

Green or chinese cabbage, cut into pieces (12 leaves)

meat minced to 300 g There was only one excursion

1 sprig of parsley 1 garlic clove Tomatoes (400 mL) diced

Tomato puree (one tablespoon) taco herbs (about a teaspoon) Corn in a small can (approximately).

cheese gratings in two hands

a sack of kidney beans weighed out to be 100 grams

Oven dish measuring 26 x 18 cm is required for this recipe.

Preparing the onion and garlic in a container after they have been chopped. After you've added the minced meat, add the taco seasonings and mix thoroughly. Make this available for free. Prepare this without cost. The tomato puree and solid shapes should be mixed in together first, then the depleted corn and kidney beans should be mixed in. Set aside for a few minutes to allow the burrito filling to thicken a bit. Bubble water will suffice for the time being.

180 degrees should be reached under the broiler. Preparation: Cut the cabbage leaves into pieces and briefly boil them (as directed by 2 or 3) in a skillet, then channel them well. Two cabbage leaves should be placed closely together, with the goal of having them cross over just a little bit. Prepare the burrito by spooning a portion of the filling onto one side of the tortilla, topping it with a little cheddar, and then carefully rolling it up. Make an effort not to push too hard. Make a second batch with the remaining cabbage leaves and filling and reheat. If they are all in the baking dish, sprinkle them with a little more cheddar cheese. For approximately 15 minutes, place the baking dish on a stovetop. Rice should be served alongside the carbs (in the event that the dish is at this point not low in carbohydrates).

Waffles made with sausage, cheese, and flour are delicious.

Complementary ingredients are as follows: (for 2 waffles)

the number of eggs is three (3)

Strained yogurt, 2 teaspoons butter (melted) 3 teaspoons

4 slices of sausage or bacon cooked at home or in a town you know and trust. Grated tongue cheese (or any other cheese you prefer): 1/2 cup

grated carrots 1 teaspoon grated carrots (optional)

one-and-a-half tablespoon almond powder (optional)

Preparation:

Prepare your waffle maker or waffle maker machine by preheating it to a high temperature. The eggs, yogurt and margarine should all be mixed together. (Optional) Miniaturize your frankfurters by chopping them into smaller pieces. Toss in a few extras to the mix. Using a wooden spoon, incorporate the ground cheddar and almonds (if using) until everything is well mixed. Delightfully grease up your waffle producer or machine. Combine two or more items and distribute them among the group. Take 5 to 10 minutes to close and not open the cover. When the timer goes off, lift the top a little to see if the food is done. Prepared with caution and served immediately after cooking. Make sure you eat your food.

Ingredients for Oopsie Bread: a loaf of bread

the number of eggs is three (3)

salt (rock/himalayan): 1 teaspoon

Cream cheese made from scratch (100 g) (you can do by passing homemade cottage cheese and butter in the food processor)

1 teaspoon of carbonate of tartar (or cream of tartar) heaped tablespoon

Preparation:

Dissolve the baking soda in a small bowl of water and add it to the eggs. As a starting point, vigorously whisk the egg whites with the carbonate and salt until extremely foamy. Then, using an electric mixer, whisk the egg yolks until they are thoroughly combined with cream cheese. With the help of a wooden spoon, gently fold in the cemented egg white froth on top of the egg yolks, ensuring that the white froths do not douse and that the mixture does not appear watery in appearance. Make an enormous plate of baking paper the size of 6 large burger buns and pour the mixture into it with the assistance of a spoon. Bake for 15 minutes at 150 degrees Celsius on a preheated stovetop.

Don't ever let anyone in through the broiler door. When the breads are toasted, remove them from the stove and leave them on the plate until they have completely cooled. Consume the food you've prepared.

Almond flour pastry with leek minced in it

30 minutes for preparation Approximately 30 minutes to prepare the dish 6 slices of bread are provided.

In this recipe, the low carb stromboli recipe from uplateanyway.com has been tweaked. Ingredients:

For the purpose of making the dough

olive oil from the Kocamaar farm (three tablespoons) cheese tongue (250 gr)

Almond flour from Kocamaar Farm, 100 g (1 cup + 4 tablespoons)

a hen (60 g)

apple cider vinegar (about a teaspoon)

12 teaspoon bicarbonate of soda (carbonate)

Garlic (either a quarter teaspoon or a small clove) To be used internally

2 tablespoons tomato paste 4 to 5 leek stalks Minced meat (100 grams)

Oil from the Kocamaar farm Cooking Instructions: Finely cleave the leek and mince the tomato glue in a skillet with olive oil. Continue cooking with its own juice after covering the pan. Consider adding a small amount of water to the mixture if it is necessary.

Add 3 tablespoons of olive oil to a medium-sized pot and add the grated cheddar cheese. On a low heat, liquefy the ground cheddar until it condenses on top of the liquid.

Pour all of the ingredients into a large mixing bowl and combine until the batter is sticky to the hand. Add the baking soda and mix until the batter is carbonate-free.

Using baking paper, create a square shape that measures * 4-10cmx10cm * Prepare your hands by soaking them in warm water. Distribute the portion of the mixture by pressing it into the surface of the pan.

Pour the batter over the leek mortar, which has been finely chopped and set aside. Using a non-stick surface, press the excess half of the dough to open it up into a square shape, which will cover the mortar. With your fingers, press the edges together. Dark seed can be added as a finishing flourish.

For 25-30 minutes, bake at 6-160°C. You can cut and serve it whenever it is ready.

Ingredients for Thai Pumpkin Soup

500g Pumpkin 400g Carrots 1 piece Spring Onion 3 EL Coconut Oil (50 G) One Small Chili, one Clove Of Garlic, and five centimeters of Ginger (30 G) 6 Thai Basil Leaves 1 piece Lime Leaf 1TL Turmeric 500ml Vegetable Stock 400ml Coconut Milk 5leaves Thai Basil 1piece Lime Leaf

Salt is highly regarded.

E.L. Soy Sauce is a type of soy sauce that is used to make a sauce that is flavored with a variety of herbs and spices.

Coconut Oil (a generous tablespoon)

Awarded Peppercorns

(1) Lime Juice (1 EL).

Preparation: Prepare the coriander leaves for serving.

The pumpkin beverage should be discontinued. It is necessary to strip the pumpkin depending on the circumstances. Take the pumpkin out of the pumpkin and put it on the scales. Carrots should be used in a similar quantity. Carrots should be peeled and sliced. Using a large knife, cut the pumpkin and carrots into huge pieces. Remove the ginger and turmeric from the pot and set them aside. Preparation: Finely cleave all of the ingredients, including the spring onion and stew.

In a small saucepan, heat the coconut oil. Fry spring onion, ginger, bean stew, turmeric, and garlic. Add carrots and pumpkin and meal without sautéing. Add soup and coconut milk, add basil and lime leaf. Heat to the point of boiling, add basil and lime leaf. Stew on a fire for around 15 minutes until the vegetables are delicate. Prick vegetables with a needle. Assuming that the vegetables sneak off effectively, it is soft.

Remove lime leaf and basil. Puree the soup with a hand blender.

Season it with soy sauce, salt, pepper, and lime juice. Present with a little coriander.

Colorful Asparagus Caprese Salad\sIngredients (4 people) (4 people)

250G tomatoes rarities

225G Mini mozzarella Topic (s) thyme

1.5 glasses STAUDT'S cocktail asparagus

Ingredients (4 people) (4 people)

2TL chopped basil

2TL chopped parsley

1 Organic Lemon (Zeste & Saft) 1toe garlic

2EL olive oil Salt

Pepper\sPreparation

For the gremolata, wash the spices, clean them, and finely slash them. Wash the natural lemon hot, rub the skin, and crush out the juice. Strip the garlic cloves and afterward slash finely. Blend the spices in with a teaspoon of lemon zing and two teaspoons of lemon juice. Add the hacked garlic clove and the olive oil, season with salt and pepper and refrigerate in the fridge.

Remove the asparagus from the glasses and serve on plates. Wash, clean, and split the tomatoes. Spread along with the small mozzarella on the asparagus. Shower with the gremolata, season with salt and pepper and topping a couple of branches of thyme. This fits impeccably with a new Focaccia.

Nutritional Information

Calories : 140.9

Protein : 9.5 g Dietary Fiber : 0.5 g Sugars : 1.3 g

Bowl of shawarma

Ingredients for the shawarma

½ kilo of fillet or beef strips in strips

A ¼ cup of avocado oil

4 cloves of garlic chopped 1 tablespoon garam masala 2 teaspoons paprika

½ teaspoon of sea salt

½ teaspoon of pepper

Ingredients for the bowl

4 cups of spinach and other vegetables of your choice (tomato, cucumber, broccoli) (tomato, cucumber, broccoli)

2 cups of white rice

tablespoon of avocado oil Sea salt and pepper to taste

A cup of cherry tomatoes and cut in half 1 cup cucumber chopped

¼ purple onion cut into thin slices

Tzatziki sauce

Ingredients for tzatziki sauce

½ cucumber peeled and finely chopped 1 cup of yogurt of coconut\scloves of garlic peeled cloves A ½ cup of fresh dill

1 tablespoon of lemon juice

½ teaspoon of salt

¼ teaspoon of pepper

Preparation

Place the cut meat in a shallow dish. Add the avocado oil and flavors. Cover it and put it in the cooler for no less than 15 minutes.

Cook the rice while the meat is marinated. Season with salt and pepper to taste.

After the meat has been marinated, sauté it in a huge skillet over medium-high hotness until it is cooked to your liking.

Arm your dishes. It begins with an underpinning of rice and adds your vegetable favorites.

To set up the tzatziki sauce, put every one of the fixings in a food processor, and blend until it has a smooth consistency. Refrigerate until used.

Cover with tzatziki sauce.

Nutritional Facts

Calories : 475.0

Protein : 41.6 g Dietary Fiber : 4.2 g

Total Fat : 13.2 g

Chapter 9

Blue corded chicken breast

For: 4 people

Preparation time: 15 minutes Cooking time: 10 minutes

Ingredients

4 chicken breasts 2 slices of ham\s4 slices of Comté cheese

100 g of bread crumbs

2 eggs

40 g of butter

Salt and pepper from the grinder

Preparing

Cut the chicken filets in their thickness, leaving the 2 sections joined. Put a large portion of a cut of ham on one side. Place a decent cut of region cheddar and close the chicken cutlet. In a plate, beat 2 eggs with a fork to make an omelet. In another plate, pour bread scraps. Plunge the chicken bosom with the ham and cheddar on the plate with the eggs and dunk in the bread scraps. Bread scraps will stick on the departure because of the eggs. Allow the blue strips to cook in the skillet in the spread for 4 to 5 minutes on each side.

Nutrition Facts

Serving Size grams (136 g) (136 g)

Serving per 1; Calories 120 cal Calories from Fat 0.00

Amount per Serving percent DV

Total Fat 1.5 g 2 percent

Total Carbohydrate 0 g 0 percent

Dietary Fiber 0 g 0 percent

Sugars 0 g\sOther Carbohydrate 0.00 g Protein 27 g

Duck breast with mirabelle plums

For: 4 people

Preparation time: 15 minutes Cooking time: 15 minutes

Ingredients

2 duck breast (or fillet) approximately 350 g each 300 g frozen Mirabelle plums (or fresh) (or fresh)

1 tsp. chicken, ground coffee 3 cl of plum brandy

50 g of cold butter

Salt and pepper from the mill

Preparation

Let the Mirabelle defrost at room temperature.

Remove some fat from the sides of the bosoms. Cut the skin in crosspieces, utilizing a sharp blade. Put them skin side in a hot skillet, without adding fat. Cook for 6 minutes on high hotness. Turn them over and cook for 4 minutes. Allow them to lay on a plate covered with aluminum foil.

Empty the oil from the skillet without cleaning it. Toss in Mirabelle plums and cook for 2 to 3 minutes while mixing. Eliminate them from the dish and keep them warm. Supplant with the lower part of poultry weakened in water and the liquor. Bring to the bubble by stripping off the cooking juices with a wooden spoon. Mix in little bits of margarine while whisking.

Slice the duck bosoms. Mix the juice in the sauce. Mix.

Arrange the cuts of fileted duck on the plates, Pour the sauce and add the mirabelles. Serve as soon as possible after preparing it.

Nutrition Facts

Calories 102 (427 kJ) (427 kJ)

Calories from fat 32

percent Daily Value 1

Total Fat 3.5g

5 percent Sat. Fat 1.1g 5 percent

Cholesterol 64mg 21 percent

Sodium 47mg 2 percent

Total Carbs. 0g 0 percent \sDietary Fiber 0g 0 percent \sProtein 16.5g

Cooking 4 portions of steamed cod

30 minutes to prepare

The great protein in the cod invigorates the digestion and fills in as a structure material for cells, muscles, chemicals, and chemicals. Important proteins additionally forestall desires and muscle breakdown.

Ingredients\sFour cod filets (à 150 g) 2 cups (four tablespoons) Lemon juice\sbars leek\stbsps. Rapeseed oil is a type of vegetable oil produced by pressing seeds of rapeseed plants.

One hundred milliliters of vegetable broth Salt\sPepper\s½ dried thyme

½ bundle chives (10 g) (10 g) One natural lemon

Preparation

2 tbsp. lemon juice should be applied to the fish filets after they have been rinsed and dried. Cut leeks into rings after they have been cleaned and washed

1 tbsp. of oil in a small saucepan over medium heat. Oil in a container, touch fish dry, sauté for 2 minutes at medium hotness. Then, at that point, turn over, add the leftover lemon juice and 50 ml of vegetable stock and cover, cook for 5-7 minutes on low heat.

Meanwhile, heat remaining oil in a pan, sauté the leek rings in medium hotness for 2 minutes, season with salt, pepper, and thyme. Cook the leek for 5 minutes on a low heat, with the remaining vegetable stock.

Meanwhile, wash the chives and dry them well before cutting them into little rolls. Wash lemon hot and cut into quarters

Season fish filets and leeks with salt and pepper, orchestrate on plates and topping with chives and lemon quarters.

Calories: 226 kcal (Nutritional Fact)

Soup with rice, potatoes and chicken

Boil 60 g of chicken with flavors for 30 minutes. Little hack 70 g of potatoes.

Then cleave 1 head of onion and broil it.

Then pour potatoes and 30 g of rice into the stock, heat up the organization for 15 minutes. Salt, put narrows leaf and leave to implant for about a large portion of an hour.

Omelet with spinach and feta

For omelet: 2 huge eggs; 1 tablespoon of milk without lactose; a spot of pepper.

Filling: 40 grams of spinach leaves; 30 grams of slashed feta cheddar; 10 gr simmered pine nuts.

Beat eggs delicately with milk and a touch of pepper. In a non-stick dish, liquefy the spread over moderate hotness until it starts to murmur. Pour in the egg blend and spread over the container to make a far round omelet. Cover with a tight-fitting top so the outer layer of the egg is practically not cooked.

Heat spinach and feta in a softly oiled dish. Put a spoonful of warmed fixings in a large portion of an omelet and cover again for 20 seconds. Eliminate the cover and sprinkle with pine nuts. Overlay the omelet in half to cover the filling.

Young potato salad with arugula

Boil youthful potatoes (4 laptops), then, at that point, add olive oil (20 gr), juice ½ lemon and a modest bunch of cleaved parsley. Let it cool.

Mix with hard-bubbled quarter-cut eggs (2 pcs).

Serve with arugula leaves (1 pack) and diced cucumber. Meat with potatoes

Prepare: 680 grams of medium-sized youthful potatoes; 1 red and 1 green ringer pepper; 500 UAH diced pork filet; 30 gr of olive oil with garlic; salt and pepper to taste.

Preheat broiler to 250 ° C. Cover the skillet with aluminum foil. In an enormous bowl, blend potatoes, peppers, meat and olive oil. Spread the combination equitably on a baking sheet.

Season with salt and pepper. Bake for 30 minutes or until the meat is prepared, and attempt the potatoes with a fork.

Ingredients: Stuffed pepper

450 gr of ground hamburger (or turkey); ½ cup pounded tomato; ¼ a glass of water; 2 medium red peppers, cut down the middle, eliminate the stem and seeds; ½ cup ground cheddar cheese.

Filling: diced tomatoes; slashed olives; destroyed green onions; coriander.

Preheat stove to 250 ° C. Fry ground hamburger in an enormous dish until cooked. Add tomato puree, water and preparing. Set the combination on the parts of pepper, dispersing it equally.

Sprinkle a little cheddar on top. Heat for 20 minutes or until pepper arrives at wanted taste. Eliminate from broiler and let cool marginally. Serve warm.

What Can You Do About Irritable Bowel Syndrome?

Women are two times as prone to be determined to have touchy entrail disorder as men.

Irritable inside condition (IBS) is a typical infection that influences 10 Australians, and two times however many ladies as men. Side effects incorporate persistent stomach torment, stoppage or the runs, and swelling. These are significant in impacting an individual's nature of life.

Many individuals utilize the term bad tempered gut disorder to depict side effects of general inside and entrail brokenness. In any case, the conclusion requires the satisfaction of authoritative and demonstrative models. ROME standards, which are known as expect that the individual experience stomach torment no less than one day seven days. Torment ought to be related with at least two of the following:

Defecation

A change in stool frequency

A change in stool shape (appearance)

The manifestation that showed up over the most recent three months started no less than a half year before the diagnosis.

If these side effects are available, tests are not needed all the time for analysis. Nonetheless, the conclusive analysis of IBS is significant on the grounds that a few manifestations, like pelvic torment, may cover with different infections like endometriosis or fiery gut sickness. Assuming you have different manifestations, a specialist might have to perform blood tests, pelvic ultrasound, endoscopy, or stool tests that prohibit comparable disorders.

Some side effects are viewed as warning "indications and ought to require further testing and master exhortation. For instance, on the off chance that you have rectal dying, weight reduction, and age north of 50 when indications start, this isn't IBS.

Causing

No single reason has been distinguished for IBS. IBS can run in families, however did you actually don't have the foggiest idea about that it's normal hereditary or due to environmental factors. A disease brought about by infections or microorganisms in a gastroenteritis area expands the gamble of creating IBS. Notwithstanding, this is generally impermanent, and the manifestations slowly improve.

People with IBS are likewise frequently Anxiety and melancholy. Research shows that youth injury can engage IBS in later life to engage certain individuals. This is on the grounds that the

digestive and cerebrum nerve signals, gastrointestinal, or stress chemicals are delivered and converse with one another through other means.

We realize that feelings can straightforwardly adjust digestive capacity. Nonetheless, concentrates on now show that inside work likewise influences feelings. An Australian review showed that for certain individuals, digestive manifestations previously showed up and, in the long run, mental indications. In any case, this isn't valid for all individuals with IBS.

What to do

Non-drug treatments ought to be thought about at first, and different treatment systems might be expected to help improve symptoms. Quality proof shows Low FODMAP diet diminishes IBS indications. FODMAPs are starches that produce abundance gas when processed. It is found in roots like onions and garlic and in natural products (or seeds) like vegetables, apples, pears, and mangoes. For best outcomes, one should begin a low FODMAP diet under the direction of an accomplished dietitian.

It is a typical confusion that individuals ought to follow a low FODMAP diet forever. Food varieties like onions found in FODMAPs are great prebiotics and advance the improvement of well disposed gastrointestinal microbes. Confine them is related with an assortment of microbes in the digestive system, immune system illnesses, and stoutness might cause underneath. This is one more justification behind a dietitian to direct individuals through the eating regimen for quite a long time and keep away from superfluous dietary restrictions.

Simple eating routine measures incorporate adding more solvent fiber to your eating regimen. This might incorporate psyllium, which might be bought as a powder from scientific experts and wellbeing shops. Insoluble fibers such as dandruff are often useless.

A probiotic preliminary could work. They can be tried for a month and afterward reconsidered by the GP, however are probably not going to be helpful whenever utilized endlessly. The activity was displayed in randomized preliminaries to further develop gut manifestations in individuals with IBS.

Managing pressure and nervousness is the way to further developing indications for some individuals. Mental medicines have been displayed in preliminaries to help manifestations more than fake treatment or different mediations. This happens particularly when the analyst is keen on IBS.

Peppermint oil can assist with diminishing stomach cramps related with IBS.

Clinical investigations, for certain individuals, digestive hypnotherapy, are just about as successful as the Low FODMAP diet. The advantages are as yet apparent in a half year. Nonetheless, hypnotherapy isn't the best thing in the world everybody, and various meetings are expected to improve symptoms. About the drugs

IBS influences the personal satisfaction however doesn't adjust an individual's gamble of sudden passing or malignant growth. In this manner, medicines ought to have a few secondary effects to be adequate. Clinical studies have shown that drugs such as peppermint oil (usually given in capsules) can reduce distressing abdominal cramps with minimal side effects. Melatonin can further develop indications on account of better rest quality when rest is uncomfortable.

The decision of prescription ought to be adjusted to every individual 's manifestations. For instance, low-portion antidepressants might be especially valuable for certain individuals with huge side effects of melancholy or tension related with IBS. Meds that decrease irritation are frequently pointless in light of the fact that they are predictable and clinically articulated aggravation isn't essential for the syndrome.

Several new ways to deal with IBS, including waste transplantation and new medications, are being attempted. Be that as it may, they all need better long haul information before they show up on the marke.

CPSIA information can be obtained
at www.ICGtesting.com
Printed in the USA
BVHW061759160822
644714BV00007BA/406